COMPLETE GUIDE TO UNDERSTANDING SPINAL FUSION SURGERY

Comprehensive Insights, Benefits, Risks, Recovery, Step-By-Step Procedures, Pain Management, And Post-Operative Care For Spondylodesis

KLEIN HOYLE

Disclaimer

The content in this book is based on the author's expertise and comprehension of the topic. The author has no affiliation or link with any corporation, business, or person. This book is meant to give general information and educational material only, and it should not be interpreted as professional medical advice. Always seek the advice of a skilled healthcare expert if you have any queries about medical issues or treatments. The author and publisher expressly disclaim any responsibility resulting directly or indirectly from the use or use of the information included in this book.

Table of Contents

ABOUT THIS BOOK

The "Complete Guide to Understanding Spinal Fusion Surgery" is an essential resource for anybody considering spinal fusion surgery or wanting thorough information on the process. From a thorough examination of spinal anatomy to insights into surgical procedures and patient experiences, this book covers everything with clarity and depth.

Chapter 1 introduces readers to the foundations of spinal fusion surgery, including its needs, advantages, and hazards. Understanding the reasoning behind the technique is critical for making sound decisions, and this chapter gives a good basis.

Chapter 2 goes into the complexities of spinal anatomy, explaining how diverse spinal diseases need fusion for support. This concept emphasizes the significance of spinal health for total well-being, which is further upon in later chapters.

Preparing for surgery is a multidimensional process, as explained in Chapter 3. From discussions with spine experts to mental and emotional preparation, every detail is painstakingly handled to ensure patients are well-informed and prepared for the treatment.

Chapter 4 investigates the surgical procedures and approaches used in spinal fusion, comparing minimally invasive treatments to classic open surgery. Readers learn about the instruments and implants utilized, as well as advances in surgical methods that improve results.

On the day of surgery, Chapter 5 gives a thorough review of what to anticipate, from pre-surgical preparations to anesthetic alternatives. Understanding these things reduces anxiety and promotes a feeling of preparation for the surgery.

Recovery is a vital step after surgery, as described in Chapter 6. From pain management measures to rehabilitation regimens, readers are led through the healing process, including a clear timeframe for returning to regular activities.

Despite its advantages, spinal fusion surgery has the potential for problems, which are discussed in Chapter 7. Readers learn to spot indicators of post-surgery issues and the significance of follow-up treatment in reducing risks.

Chapter 8 discusses the long-term prognosis and lifestyle modifications after surgery. Rehabilitation activities and lifestyle changes are addressed, allowing patients to make proactive efforts toward spinal health.

Patient anecdotes and experiences recounted in Chapter 9 provide essential insights, emphasizing the difficulties encountered throughout rehabilitation and the need for a support system. These stories connect with readers, offering encouragement and insight.

Finally, Chapter 10 investigates future discoveries and breakthroughs in spinal surgery, providing optimism for improved treatment alternatives. Emerging technology and possible future therapies highlight the necessity of continued research and innovation for improving surgical results.

Finally, "Complete Guide to Understanding Spinal Fusion Surgery" is a complete and powerful resource for patients, caregivers, and healthcare professionals alike, providing essential insights and assistance at each step of the surgical process.

CHAPTER 1

Introduction To Spinal Fusion Surgery

What Is Spinal Fusion Surgery?

Spinal fusion surgery is a treatment for connecting two or more vertebrae in the spine. It is often used to treat degenerative disc disease, spinal instability, spinal abnormalities such as scoliosis, and vertebral fractures. The objective is to stabilize the spine and relieve discomfort by forming a solid mass of bone between the vertebrae.

When Is It Necessary?

Spinal fusion surgery is required when conservative therapies such as medicine, physical therapy, or injections fail to alleviate symptoms or when the spine is severely unstable or injured.

Serious back discomfort, spinal stenosis, ruptured discs, or spinal fractures may need spinal fusion surgery.

Benefits And Risks Of The Procedure

Benefits:

• Pain Relief: Spinal fusion surgery may provide great pain relief. The operation may relieve movement-related discomfort by stabilizing the spine and limiting mobility in the afflicted region.

• Vertebral fusion improves spinal stability, preventing future injury and ensuring adequate alignment.

• Spinal fusion surgery may restore lost function or prevent future degeneration in some diseases, such as spinal abnormalities.

Risks:

• Operative procedures carry the risk of infection at the operative site.

• Surgery might raise the chance of blood clots developing in the legs, which can be life-threatening if they reach the lungs.

• Surgery may cause nerve injury, resulting in weakness, numbness, or paralysis.

• Failed fusion might cause discomfort and need extra surgery.

Overview Of The Surgical Process

Preoperative Preparation:

Before surgery, you will have a full assessment, including imaging tests such as X-rays or MRI scans to determine the amount of spinal injury. Your medical staff will advise you on how to prepare for the operation, which may involve fasting and quitting certain medicines.

Anesthesia:

During the operation, you will be given a general anesthetic to keep you asleep and pain-free. In rare situations, the surgeon may additionally use a local anesthetic to numb the region around the spine.

Incision:

The surgeon will create an incision in your back, often over the damaged portion of the spine. The size and placement of the incision may vary according to the problem being treated.

Bone Grafts:

To encourage fusion, bone graft material is inserted between the vertebrae. This may be sourced from your own body (autograft), a donor (allograft), or synthetic materials.

Fusion:

The surgeon will use screws, rods, or plates to keep the vertebrae in place while the bone transplant cures and fused them. This hardware ensures stability and support during the healing process.

Once the fusion is complete, the incision is sutured or stapled closed, and a bandage is put on to preserve the wound.

Following surgery, you will be carefully observed in the recovery area before being transported to your hospital room. Your postoperative treatment plan will include pain management, physical therapy, and activity limitations to promote a smooth recovery and optimum spinal repair.

CHAPTER 2

Understanding Spinal Anatomy

Basic Anatomy Of The Spine

The spine, or vertebral column, is an important component in the human body that supports, stretches, and protects the spinal cord. It is made up of 33 vertebrae organized into five regions: cervical (neck), thoracic (upper back), lumbar (lower back), sacral, and coccygeal (tailbone). Each vertebra has a distinct structure, including a body, arch, processes, and foramina.

The cervical spine consists of seven vertebrae that support the head and allow for neck mobility. The thoracic spine, which consists of twelve vertebrae, links to the rib cage and stabilizes the upper body. The lumbar spine, which consists of five vertebrae, carries the greatest weight and allows for mobility in the lower back.

The sacral and coccygeal areas are joined to create the base of the spine, which supports the pelvis.

Intervertebral discs connect each vertebra and function as shock absorbers while also allowing for spinal flexibility. The discs have a strong outer layer (annulus fibrosus) and a gel-like inner core (nucleus pulposus). The vertebral canal contains the spinal cord, which is protected by the spine's bone components.

Common Spinal Conditions Requiring Fusion

Several spinal problems may need spinal fusion surgery to relieve pain and stabilize the spine. One prevalent illness is degenerative disc disease, in which the intervertebral discs degrade over time, causing pain, stiffness, and decreased mobility. Spinal fusion may help restore stability and alleviate discomfort by fusing two or more vertebrae and removing mobility from the afflicted section.

Other disorders include spinal stenosis, which occurs when the spinal canal narrows and compresses the spinal cord or nerves, resulting in pain, numbness, and weakness in the arms or legs. Spinal fusion surgery may also help with spondylolisthesis, a condition in which one vertebra slides forward over the one below it, by stabilizing the spine and relieving nerve strain.

Traumatic injuries to the spine, such as fractures or dislocations, may need fusion to realign and stabilize the afflicted vertebrae. Furthermore, some spinal abnormalities, such as scoliosis or kyphosis, may be repaired by spinal fusion surgery to enhance spine alignment and function.

Spinal Fusion Helps To Stabilize The Spine

Spinal fusion surgery seeks to stabilize the spine by forming a strong link between two or more vertebrae, minimizing excessive movement and alleviating discomfort.

During the operation, the surgeon will remove the injured intervertebral disc and insert a bone transplant between the neighboring vertebrae. The bone transplant may be extracted from the patient's body (autograft) or a donor (allograft).

Over time, the bone transplant promotes the formation of new bone tissue, uniting the vertebrae into a single, solid structure. Metal implants, such as screws, rods, or cages, may be utilized to enhance support and stability throughout the fusion process. These implants aid in maintaining appropriate alignment and encourage vertebral fusion.

As the fusion cures, the treated segment becomes immovable, relieving discomfort and avoiding further injury to the spinal nerves or surrounding tissues. Physical therapy and rehabilitation may be needed after surgery to enhance strength, flexibility, and general spinal health.

Spinal Health Is Important For Overall Well-Being

Maintaining spinal health is critical for general well-being since the spine supports the body, protects the spinal cord, and allows mobility. A strong spine promotes good posture, balance, and mobility, lowering the chance of injury and chronic discomfort.

Good posture, frequent exercise, and a healthy weight may all help prevent and enhance spinal health. Avoiding activities that strain the spine, such as heavy lifting or extended sitting, may help to lower the risk of injury and degenerative disorders.

Individuals may make more educated judgments regarding their spinal health and treatment options if they understand the fundamental architecture of the spine, prevalent spinal diseases, and the function of spinal fusion in spinal stabilization. Prioritizing spinal health via preventative measures and adequate medical treatment may lead to an improved quality of life and overall well-being.

CHAPTER 3

Preparing For Surgery

Consult With A Spine Specialist

Before having spinal fusion surgery, speak with a spine expert. This consultation serves several functions. First, it enables the expert to assess your unique situation and decide if spinal fusion is the best treatment choice for you. During this session, the doctor will evaluate your medical history, perform a physical examination, and prescribe further tests such as X-rays or MRI scans to better analyze the health of your spine.

The consultation also gives you the chance to ask any questions you may have concerning the process. You may talk about the risks and advantages of spinal fusion, as well as any other treatment alternatives that may be available.

It is important to communicate openly and honestly with your expert so that you completely understand what to anticipate before, during, and after surgery.

Furthermore, the meeting enables the professional to develop a unique treatment plan based on your specific requirements. They will explain the surgical approach to be employed, the estimated recovery time, and any post-operative care needs. By the conclusion of the session, you should be confident and informed about your choice to have spinal fusion surgery.

Medical Tests And Evaluations Before Surgery

Various medical tests and assessments will be performed before spinal fusion surgery to verify that you are in good enough health for the operation. These tests are used to discover any underlying medical issues that may complicate the procedure or influence your recovery.

Blood tests, urinalysis, and an electrocardiogram (ECG) are common medical tests performed before spinal fusion surgery to examine your general health and detect any underlying medical diseases such as diabetes, renal disease, or heart problems. Furthermore, imaging tests like as X-rays, MRI scans, or CT scans may be used to offer comprehensive pictures of your spine and assist the surgeon in planning the surgical approach.

Depending on your age and medical history, you may also need to have a comprehensive physical examination, which will include tests of your cardiovascular and pulmonary systems. These examinations are necessary to guarantee that you can withstand the anesthetic and surgical stress.

Pre-Surgery Instructions And Lifestyle Adjustments

Your healthcare team will provide you with pre-surgical instructions in the weeks before your spinal fusion surgery.

These guidelines are intended to help you improve your health and prepare for the surgery. Common pre-surgery instructions might include:

• Medication management: Your healthcare practitioner may advise you to discontinue certain drugs, such as blood thinners, before surgery to lessen the risk of bleeding during the operation.

• Smoking cessation: If you smoke, it may be recommended to cease several weeks before surgery. Smoking may impair the body's capacity to recover, increasing the likelihood of problems during and after surgery.

• Maintaining a balanced diet before surgery may aid in recovery. To encourage tissue regeneration and healing, your healthcare professional may prescribe that you consume more protein, vitamins, and minerals.

• Regular exercise and physical activity before surgery may strengthen muscles and improve general fitness, thereby aiding recovery. However, it is critical to avoid high-impact activities or workouts that may worsen your spinal condition.

Follow these pre-surgical guidelines and make any required lifestyle changes to help achieve the best potential result from your spinal fusion surgery.

Mental And Emotional Preparedness For Procedure

Preparing for spinal fusion surgery requires not only physical but also mental and emotional preparation. Any medical operation may be intimidating, but making efforts to prepare psychologically and emotionally can help reduce worry and create a good attitude.

One important component of mental preparation is to educate oneself about the surgery and what to anticipate throughout the recovery period. This may include studying the operation, consulting with your healthcare provider, and networking with others who have experienced comparable surgeries. Understanding the reasoning behind the procedure and the predicted results may assist in reducing concerns and uncertainty.

It's also critical to devise coping skills to deal with any worry or tension that may arise before the operation. Deep breathing exercises, meditation, and visualization exercises are all examples of relaxation methods. Maintaining open contact with your healthcare staff and loved ones may also be beneficial and reassuring at this time.

Finally, exercising self-care and participating in activities that provide comfort and relaxation may help you achieve emotional well-being. Prioritizing self-care, whether by spending time with loved ones, engaging in a favorite pastime, or just taking time for yourself, may help you feel more resilient and prepared for the difficulties that lie ahead.

CHAPTER 4

Surgical Techniques And Approaches

Different Methods Of Spinal Fusion Surgery

Spinal fusion surgery takes several forms, each suited to unique spinal problems and patient requirements. The two main procedures are posterior and anterior fusion. In posterior fusion, the surgeon approaches the spine from behind, while in anterior fusion, they approach it from the front. These approaches have additional subdivisions, such as:

1. **Posterior Fusion Techniques:**

• Pedicle screw fixation includes inserting screws into vertebral pedicles and attaching them to rods to support the spine.

• The transforaminal lumbar interbody fusion (TLIF) procedure includes removing the disc between two vertebrae and connecting them using bone transplants.

• Posterolateral gutter fusion involves placing bone grafts along the back of the spine to promote vertebral union.

2. Anterior Fusion Techniques:

• The anterior cervical discectomy and fusion (ACDF) procedure removes a damaged disc from the cervical spine and fuses the neighboring vertebrae.

• Anterior lumbar interbody fusion (ALIF) is similar to TLIF but accessible from the front, providing greater access to the lumbar spine.

3. Lateral Fusion Techniques:

• XLIF surgery includes entering the spine by a tiny incision in the patient's side, avoiding major muscles, and fusing vertebral bodies.

Each treatment has benefits and is selected depending on the location and severity of the spinal disease, the patient's anatomy, and the surgeon's preferences. Discussing these choices with your surgeon can assist in determining the best course of action for your particular circumstance.

Minimally Invasive Vs. Traditional Open Surgery

The progress of spinal fusion surgery has resulted in the development of minimally invasive procedures, which have various advantages over conventional open surgery:

Minimal Invasive Surgery (MIS):

• MIS uses fewer incisions than typical open surgery, reducing tissue damage and blood loss.

• MIS allows surgeons to avoid cutting or detaching muscles, resulting in speedier recovery and less postoperative discomfort.

• Patients who undergo MIS had shorter hospital stays and a faster return to regular activities compared to standard open surgery.

• Enhanced visualization: MIS procedures use specialized equipment and imaging technology to improve surgical site visibility, even with tiny incisions.

Traditional open surgery:

• Traditional open surgery involves wider incisions to reach the spine, which may cause tissue stress and prolong healing periods.

• Traditional surgery may cause substantial muscle damage, resulting in increased discomfort and longer recovery.

• Patients having conventional open surgery may need extended hospital stays for postoperative monitoring and rehabilitation.

The decision between minimally invasive and standard open surgery is based on the patient's general health, the intricacy of the spinal problem, and the surgeon's skill. While MIS has several benefits, not all patients are candidates for this technique. Your surgeon will analyze your situation and propose the best surgical procedure for you.

Instruments And Implants Used During The Procedure

Instrumentation and implants are critical for spine stabilization during fusion surgery. These implants serve to keep the vertebrae in appropriate alignment and aid the fusion process. Common kinds of apparatus and implants used in spinal fusion surgery are:

1. Pedicle Screws:

• Pedicle screws stabilize and support spinal bones during fusion.

They are often used in tandem with rods to form a structure that keeps the spine in the appropriate position.

2. Rods and plates:

• Rods and plates link pedicle screws and give spinal support. They are usually composed of metal alloys such as titanium or stainless steel and are available in a variety of sizes and forms to fit the diverse spinal architecture.

3. Interbody cages:

• Interbody cages are implanted between vertebrae to restore disc height, relieve nerve compression, and encourage fusion. These cages are often filled with bone graft material to aid in the fusion of neighboring vertebrae.

4. Bone Grafts:
• Bone transplants promote bone development and fusion between vertebral bones.

They may be taken from the patient's own body (autograft) or donors (allograft). In certain circumstances, synthetic bone transplant alternatives may be employed.

5. BMPs are classified as bone morphogenetic proteins.

• BMPs are biological agents that promote bone growth and expedite fusion. They are often used in combination with bone grafts to improve fusion rates, particularly in difficult situations or when a considerable volume of bone graft material is needed.

The surgeon's inclination and expertise, as well as the patient's spinal anatomy, and the kind and location of the spinal problem, all influence the choice of apparatus and implants. Your surgeon will explain the many alternatives to you and propose the best devices for your unique situation.

Advancements In Surgical Technique

Advances in surgical methods have transformed spinal fusion surgery, resulting in better results, fewer problems, and shorter recovery periods. Some significant advances include:

1. Navigation systems:

• Computer-assisted navigation devices improve spinal fusion surgery by providing real-time guidance for accurate implant placement and spine alignment. This technique improves surgical precision while lowering the risk of complications.

2. Robotics:

• Robotic-assisted surgery improves doctors' accuracy and control during difficult spinal surgeries. Robotic systems combine enhanced imaging and robotic arms to let surgeons navigate the spine and place implants with unprecedented precision.

3. Minimally Invasive Techniques:

• Refinements in surgical equipment, imaging technology, and procedures are driving the evolution of minimally invasive methods. These innovations enable fewer incisions, less tissue stress, and shorter recovery periods than conventional open surgery.

4. Biologics:

• Biologic medicines such as bone morphogenetic proteins (BMPs) and growth factors are being employed to improve bone fusion and healing. These biologics enhance the body's healing systems, resulting in quicker and stronger fusion.

5. Patient-specific implants:

• 3D printing technology enables personalized implants based on individual anatomy. These bespoke implants provide a superior fit and alignment, lowering the risk of implant-related problems and increasing long-term results.

Using these improvements, surgeons may provide patients with safer, more effective, and less intrusive treatment choices for a variety of spinal diseases. However, it is important to realize that not all patients will benefit from these technologies, and surgical choices should be made on an individual basis after a thorough examination of the patient's specific requirements and circumstances.

CHAPTER 5

Day Of Surgery

What To Expect On The Day Of Surgery

The day of your spinal fusion surgery is likely to be filled with a range of feelings, from excitement to anxiety. Knowing what to anticipate helps alleviate some of those emotions. Typically, you will arrive at the hospital or surgical facility several hours before your planned procedure. This permits the medical staff to finalize any necessary preparations and confirm that everything is in order.

After checking in, you will be brought to a pre-operative area to change into a hospital gown. Nurses will evaluate your medical history, take your vital signs, and begin an IV line for fluids and drugs. You may also meet with your surgeon and anesthesiologist to address any last-minute questions or concerns.

Pre-Surgical Preparations At The Hospital

Before the procedure, various critical preparations will be made at the hospital. These include validating your identification and the intended procedure, making sure all relevant equipment is present and operational, and double-checking any pre-operative tests or imaging studies.

Additionally, you may be given drugs to help you relax and avoid discomfort or infection. Depending on your medical history and the specifics of your operation, you may be required to undergo additional tests or procedures, such as blood tests or X-rays.

Anesthesia Options And Their Effects

Anesthesia is an important element of spinal fusion surgery because it keeps you comfortable and pain-free during the treatment.

Depending on the intricacy of the operation and your specific requirements, a variety of anesthetic techniques may be employed.

• General anesthesia is the most often used for spinal fusion surgery. It entails providing drugs that cause unconsciousness, enabling you to sleep during the process. Anesthesiologists will constantly monitor your breathing and other important processes while you are under general anesthesia.

• Some surgeons may use localized anesthetic, which numbs a particular area of the body while keeping the patient awake. This may be coupled with a sedative to help you relax during surgery.

• Local anesthesia includes administering numbing medicine directly to the operative site. While this may be utilized for certain minimally invasive procedures, it is less usual for spinal fusion surgery since it requires deeper anesthesia.

A Brief Overview Of The Surgical Process

The surgical team will begin the spinal fusion surgery when you have been anesthetized and correctly positioned on the operating table. The individual strategy and procedures used by your surgeon will determine the exact processes needed, but in general, the process comprises the following:

1. **Incision:** Your surgeon will create an incision over the affected portion of the spine, which is usually in the lower back or the neck.

2. **Exposure:** The muscles and tissues that surround the spine will be gently pulled aside to provide access to the vertebrae.

3. **Bone Graft Preparation:** If bone graft material is required, it will be collected from another region of your body or received from a donor and prepared for implantation.

4. Fusion: Your surgeon will carefully remove any damaged or diseased tissue from the spine before inserting the bone graft material between the afflicted vertebrae. Metal implants, such as screws, rods, or cages, may also be used to support the spine and encourage fusion.

5. Closure: Once the bone graft is in place and the spine has been stabilized, the incision will be closed with sutures or staples and a sterile bandage will be placed.

After the procedure, you will be sent to a recovery room where medical personnel will carefully monitor your status as you awaken from anesthesia. Once you are awake and stable, you will be transferred to a hospital room or released home to begin your recuperation.

CHAPTER 6

Recovery Process

Immediate Post-Surgery Care At The Hospital

Immediate post-operative care is essential after spinal fusion surgery to ensure a smooth recovery. In the hospital, healthcare workers will continuously monitor you to guarantee your safety and comfort. You will most likely wake up in the recovery room, also known as the post-anesthesia care unit (PACU), just after surgery. Nurses will check your vital signs and treat any acute postoperative pain or discomfort.

Your healthcare staff will explain how to move safely and comfortably. They may utilize strategies like as turning you on your side or utilizing a customized bed to maintain your spine in good alignment. Pain management will be a top concern at this time, and you will most likely be given medicine to relieve any pain.

As you recover from anesthesia, you may feel nauseated or groggy. This is typical and should improve with time. Nurses will monitor your drug response and assist you manage any adverse effects that may occur.

Depending on your procedure and particular requirements, you may be in the hospital for a few days to a week. During this period, your healthcare team will continue to evaluate your progress, manage your pain, and provide advice on activities and mobility.

Pain Management Strategies

Pain management is an important part of the healing process after spinal fusion surgery. Your healthcare team will collaborate with you to create a pain management strategy that is specifically customized to your requirements and preferences.

Immediately after surgery, you will most likely be given pain medicine by intravenous (IV) drip or injection. Opioids for severe pain may be prescribed, as well as non-opioid treatments such as acetaminophen or anti-inflammatory drugs to alleviate discomfort.

As you go from the hospital to home, your pain management strategy may include oral drugs like prescription opioids or over-the-counter pain remedies. It's critical to closely follow your healthcare provider's recommendations and discuss any concerns or changes in your pain levels.

Aside from medicine, alternative pain management measures may include cold packs or heat therapy, relaxation techniques such as deep breathing or meditation, and positioning techniques to alleviate tension on the surgical site.

Rehabilitation And Physical Therapy

Rehabilitation and physical therapy are essential in the healing process after spinal fusion surgery. These programs are intended to help you rebuild strength, flexibility, and mobility in your spine and surrounding muscles.

Your healthcare team will collaborate with you to create a tailored rehabilitation plan based on your unique requirements and objectives. This might include exercises to enhance core strength, flexibility, and posture, as well as activities to progressively build endurance and stamina.

Physical therapy sessions may begin in the hospital immediately after surgery and continue as outpatient care after you are released. During these sessions, a physical therapist will walk you through exercises and strategies to safely improve your strength and mobility.

Attend all planned physical therapy visits and attentively follow your therapist's recommendations. Consistency and attention to your rehabilitation program might help you heal faster and with fewer difficulties.

Timeline For Recovery And Returning To Normal Activities

The recovery period and return to regular activities after spinal fusion surgery vary based on the kind of surgery, the amount of the fusion, and individual characteristics such as general health and fitness level.

In general, you should anticipate a progressive healing period lasting from weeks to months. Immediately after surgery, you should concentrate on rest and healing, gradually increasing your activity level as tolerated.

You may feel some pain and have limited mobility for the first several weeks following surgery. Your healthcare team will advise you on when it is safe to resume activities such as driving, lifting, and returning to work.

As you proceed through the healing process, you will collaborate closely with your healthcare team to track your progress and alter your activity level as necessary. Physical therapy and rehabilitation can help you restore strength, flexibility, and function.

It is important to be patient and listen to your body throughout the rehabilitation process. Pushing yourself too hard or resuming regular activities too soon might raise the risk of problems and slow recovery. Follow your healthcare provider's advice and instructions to ensure a safe and successful recovery.

CHAPTER 7

Possible Complications And Risks

Common Complications Of Spinal Fusion Surgery

Spinal fusion surgery, like any other surgical operation, has inherent risks and problems. It is essential to be aware of these possibilities to make sound choices and appropriately prepare for the surgery. Common consequences of spinal fusion surgery include infection, hemorrhage, nerve injury, and fusion failure.

Infection is one of the most serious problems after spinal fusion surgery. Despite the measures used in the operating room, there is always a possibility of bacterial contamination, which may lead to infection at the surgery site. Infection symptoms may include fever, discomfort, edema, and redness around the incision site. If any indications of infection are observed, get medical assistance right once.

Another possible risk is bleeding, which is quite uncommon. Excessive bleeding during or after surgery may need further treatments for management and may result in problems such as blood clots or hematoma development. Close monitoring by the surgical team is required to appropriately control bleeding and avoid complications.

Nerve injury is a danger in all spinal surgeries, including fusion operations. Nerve damage may cause temporary or permanent sensory or motor abnormalities, including weakness, numbness, and pain in the afflicted regions. Surgeons make efforts to reduce the danger of nerve injury during surgery, but it is still a possible consequence that patients should know about.

Failure of fusion, also known as pseudoarthrosis, occurs when the bones do not join adequately after surgery. This may cause chronic discomfort and instability in the spine, necessitating multiple procedures to resolve. Smoking, poor bone quality, and inappropriate surgical technique may all lead to fusion failure. Close monitoring and follow-up with the surgeon are required to discover indications of pseudoarthrosis early and act effectively.

Strategies To Prevent Complications

While problems cannot always be avoided, several techniques may assist to reduce the risk and improve results after spinal fusion surgery. Preoperative optimization, which includes treating any underlying medical issues such as diabetes or obesity, may lower the risk of complications before and after surgery.

During the surgical operation, rigorous attention to detail and the use of sterile methods may help avoid infections and minimize the risk of bleeding. To reduce tissue stress and promote healing, surgeons may utilize antibiotics as a preventative measure as well as new surgical technology such as minimally invasive procedures.

Postoperative care is equally crucial in avoiding problems. Patients are often recommended to follow stringent activity limitations and wound care procedures to reduce the risk of infection and promote normal healing. Physical therapy and rehabilitation are critical for enhancing healing and lowering the risk of problems like nerve injury or fusion failure.

Signs Of Post-Surgical Complications

Patients must be cautious and informed of possible consequences after spinal fusion surgery. Any odd symptoms or changes should be reported immediately to the medical staff for investigation and treatment. Signs of postoperative problems may include:

• Experiencing unexpected pain or discomfort after surgery.

• Swelling, redness, or warmth around the surgery site may suggest infection.

• Persistent numbness, weakness, or tingling in the arms, legs, or other places may indicate nerve injury.

• Problems with bowel or bladder function may suggest nerve compression or other issues.

• Failure to progress in rehabilitation or increased symptoms may indicate a problem with fusion or other concerns that need to be addressed.

Early detection and action are critical for successfully treating postoperative complications and enhancing outcomes.

Importance Of Follow-Up Care With Surgeon

Follow-up care with the surgeon is critical for tracking recovery progress, identifying any issues early on, and addressing any concerns or questions that may emerge.

Patients are often scheduled for follow-up sessions at regular intervals after surgery to check healing, monitor fusion progress, and change treatment plans as required.

During follow-up visits, the surgeon will do physical exams, examine imaging results such as X-rays or MRIs, and discuss any complaints or changes in health status with the patient. Based on the results, the surgeon may suggest further therapies, such as physical therapy, medication changes, or more imaging investigations.

Regular contact with the surgical team ensures that any concerns or complications are handled swiftly, lowering the risk of long-term problems and improving recovery results. Patients should stick to the specified follow-up plan and be proactive in reporting any concerns or changes in symptoms between consultations.

Understanding the potential complications of spinal fusion surgery, implementing prevention strategies, monitoring for signs of post-surgery issues, and prioritizing follow-up care with the surgeon are critical steps in achieving successful outcomes and minimizing risks for patients undergoing this procedure.

CHAPTER 8

Long-Term Prospects And Lifestyle Changes

Long-Term Results Of Spinal Fusion Surgery

After having spinal fusion surgery, it is critical to understand the long-term implications on your health. While the surgery's goal is to relieve pain and stabilize the spine, you should evaluate how it may affect your everyday life in the future.

Stability and Pain Relief

The main purpose of spinal fusion surgery is to stabilize the spine and relieve pain. Over time, many patients report great improvement from the problems that prompted them to seek surgery in the first place. The operation attempts to limit excessive movement, which may cause pain and discomfort, by fusing the afflicted vertebrae. While it may take some time for the fusion to properly set and the surrounding tissues to recover, patients often report that their discomfort progressively decreases in the months after surgery.

While spinal fusion surgery may help to stabilize the spine, it may restrict your range of motion in the afflicted region. This limitation in mobility is usually more obvious immediately after surgery, as your body adapts to the alterations. However, with adequate therapy and exercise, many people may retain a high degree of mobility over time. It's critical to collaborate with your healthcare team to create a rehabilitation plan that meets your requirements and objectives.

Spinal fusion surgery, like any other surgical operation, has possible problems that might have an impact on your long-term prognosis.

Infection, nerve injury, and fusion failure are all possible complications. While these consequences are uncommon, it is important to be aware of the risks and strictly adhere to your healthcare provider's advice to reduce them.

Overall Quality of Life

Many patients find that spinal fusion surgery significantly improves their overall quality of life. By lowering pain and enhancing spine stability, the operation enables people to resume activities they may have avoided earlier owing to discomfort. However, it is important to have reasonable expectations regarding the results of surgery and to be patient throughout the recuperation period. After spinal fusion surgery, many patients may resume an active and happy lifestyle with time and effort in therapy.

Rehabilitation Exercises To Maintain Spinal Health#

Rehabilitation activities are an important element of the healing process after spinal fusion surgery. These exercises aim to strengthen the muscles around the spine, increase flexibility, and enhance general spinal health. Incorporating these exercises into your everyday routine will assist in ensuring a successful recovery and lower your risk of future spine problems.

Core Strengthening

Core strengthening exercises are especially helpful following spinal fusion surgery because they support the spine and relieve stress on the joined vertebrae. These exercises work the muscles in the belly, lower back, and pelvis, helping to enhance stability and posture. Planks, bridges, and abdominal crunches are all workouts that strengthen the core. It is critical to begin cautiously and progressively raise the intensity of these workouts as your strength develops.

Flexibility exercises

Maintaining spinal flexibility is also critical for avoiding future spine problems and lowering the chance of injury. Stretching exercises may assist increase spinal flexibility and range of motion, making everyday tasks more comfortable. Stretches that target the muscles of the back, hips, and hamstrings are very beneficial following surgery. Flexibility exercises include sitting spinal twists, hamstring stretches, and cat-cow stretches.

Aerobic exercise

Aerobic activity, in addition to strength and flexibility training, is critical for long-term health and well-being after spinal fusion surgery. Walking, swimming, and cycling are all good ways to enhance cardiovascular fitness and support weight control, which is beneficial for minimizing spine strain. Begin with low-impact exercises, gradually increasing the intensity as your fitness improves.

Aim for at least 30 minutes of aerobic activity most days of the week, as advised by healthcare specialists.

Posture Correction

Poor posture may increase pre-existing pain and discomfort in the spine. After spinal fusion surgery, it is critical to monitor your posture and make modifications as required to ensure optimal alignment. Maintain excellent posture throughout the day by sitting up straight, keeping your shoulders relaxed, and avoiding slouching or curving your back. You may also find it beneficial to employ supporting furnishings, such as ergonomic chairs or cushions, to aid in maintaining excellent posture when sitting or lying down.

Lifestyle Modifications To Prevent Future Spine Issues

In addition to rehabilitative activities, lifestyle changes may help prevent future spine problems and improve overall spinal health.

By adopting healthy practices into your everyday routine, you may lower your chance of injury and extend the advantages of spinal fusion surgery over time.

Maintain a healthy weight

Excess weight may put pressure on the spine, increasing the likelihood of developing problems like herniated discs or degenerative disc degeneration. Maintaining a healthy weight via a balanced diet and regular exercise may lessen the strain on your spine and lower your chances of issues. Aim for a diet heavy in fruits, vegetables, lean proteins, and whole grains, while limiting your consumption of processed meals, sugary snacks, and high-fat foods.

Practice proper lifting techniques

Improper lifting methods may strain the spine's muscles and ligaments, increasing the risk of injury or worsening pre-existing spine disorders.

When lifting large things, always bend at the knees and maintain your back straight, utilizing the muscles in your legs and buttocks to propel the action. Avoid twisting or jerking activities, and utilize lifting belts or braces as needed to give additional spine support.

Use ergonomic equipment

Ergonomic equipment may assist minimize spine strain while also increasing overall comfort and productivity. Purchase ergonomic furniture and accessories for your home and office, such as adjustable seats, standing workstations, and supporting pillows. To decrease neck strain, position your computer display at eye level, and during extended phone conversations, use a headset or loudspeaker rather than cradling the phone between your ear and shoulder.

Practice Stress Management
Chronic stress may cause muscular strain and worsen spine problems including back pain or muscle spasms.

Include stress-relieving activities in your routine, such as meditation, deep breathing exercises, or yoga. Make time for hobbies and activities that make you happy and relaxed, and emphasize self-care techniques like getting enough sleep and taking frequent breaks during the day.

Follow-Up Appointments And Monitoring After Surgery

Following spinal fusion surgery, you should schedule frequent follow-up consultations with your healthcare practitioner to check your progress and address any issues. These sessions enable your healthcare team to evaluate your healing process, look for symptoms of problems, and change your treatment plan as required to achieve the best possible result.

Post-operative Care

Following surgery, you may need specialist care to help with pain management, wound healing, and rehabilitation. Your healthcare team will provide you with advice on how to care for your incision, manage discomfort, and gradually increase your activity level while you recuperate. It is critical that you carefully follow these directions and notify your healthcare practitioner if you have any unexpected symptoms or consequences.

Monitoring Fusion Progress

One of the primary goals of follow-up consultations after spinal fusion surgery is to track the progression of the fusion process. Your healthcare practitioner may use imaging tests, such as X-rays or CT scans, to examine the stability of the fused vertebrae and confirm that the fusion is developing as planned. Depending on your specific needs, follow-up consultations may be planned at regular intervals over many months or years to assess long-term fusion success.

Addressing Complications

In certain circumstances, difficulties may emerge after spinal fusion surgery, necessitating further intervention or therapy. Infections, hardware failures, and chronic discomfort are examples of such difficulties. If you notice any troubling symptoms or consequences, you should call your healthcare professional immediately to discuss your management and treatment options.

Rehabilitation and Support

Follow-up sessions are also a chance to address your continuing rehabilitation and support requirements while you recover from surgery. Your healthcare provider may provide advice on suitable workouts, lifestyle changes, and techniques for dealing with any chronic symptoms or limits. They may also refer you to other resources and support services as required to assist you meet your long-term spinal health and general well-being objectives.

CHAPTER 9

Patients' Stories And Experiences

Challenges During Recovery: How They Were Overcome

Recovering after spinal fusion surgery may be difficult, both physically and emotionally. Patients must recognize these problems and how to overcome them to have a more successful recovery.

Physical challenges:

1. Pain Management: Pain is a typical problem after spinal fusion surgery. Initially, patients may feel pain at the surgery site and in the surrounding muscles. However, with prescribed pain medicines and enough rest, this discomfort may be properly controlled. Physical therapy and mild activities, as prescribed by healthcare specialists, may also help relieve soreness gradually.

2. Limited Mobility: Following surgery, patients may find it difficult to move freely due to stiffness and discomfort. It is critical to follow the surgeon's post-operative recommendations and gradually raise exercise levels as tolerated. Using assistive aids like walkers or canes, as prescribed by the medical team, can help with movement throughout the rehabilitation process.

3. Fatigue: Surgery and the recovery process may cause feelings of exhaustion and low energy levels. Patients should emphasize rest and give their bodies time to recuperate. Balanced intervals of activity and proper rest periods are critical for good fatigue management.

4. Incision Care: Taking care of the surgical incision is essential for preventing infection and promoting recovery. Patients should follow their healthcare team's wound care guidelines, such as keeping the incision clean and dry and avoiding activities that may interfere with the healing process.

Emotional Challenges:

1. Emotional Adjustment: Recovering following spinal fusion surgery may be emotionally taxing, particularly if the patient's mobility or lifestyle changes. It is common to experience a variety of emotions, such as annoyance, worry, and even despair. Connecting with a support system, such as family, friends, or a therapist, may help you cope emotionally at this time.

2. Fear of Recurrence or Complications: Some patients may be concerned about the prospect of recurrent spinal disorders or surgical complications. Any concerns should be communicated to the healthcare staff, and post-operative examinations should be scheduled regularly. Education about the procedure and its possible effects might also help to reduce worries and anxiety.

3. Dependence on Others: In the early stages of rehabilitation, patients may need help with everyday tasks such as bathing, dressing, or home duties.

Some people who are used to being self-sufficient may find this reliance on others difficult. Accepting assistance from family members or caregivers, on the other hand, is critical for a good recovery.

Overcoming Challenges:

1. Maintaining open and honest contact with healthcare practitioners, family, and friends is critical throughout the healing process. Expressing concerns or asking questions might help to handle problems more effectively and ensure that the required assistance is delivered.

2. **Patience and Persistence:** Recovery after spinal fusion surgery is a long process that demands patience and perseverance. It is critical for patients to establish realistic goals and appreciate minor triumphs along the road. Many obstacles may be overcome with patience and commitment to the healing process.

3. **Using Support Systems:** Having a strong support system in place, including family, friends, and

healthcare experts, may significantly improve the rehabilitation process. Lean on loved ones for emotional support, and don't be afraid to seek medical advice and help as required.

Insights And Advice From Patients To Others Preparing For Surgery

Learning from the experiences of people who have had spinal fusion surgery may give significant insights and guidance to those preparing for the treatment. Below are some typical themes and suggestions from patients:

1. **Educate Yourself:** Learn about the surgical process, including its risks, advantages, and anticipated results. Understanding what to anticipate might help reduce anxiety and psychologically prepare for the operation and recovery period.

2. **Follow Pre-Operative Instructions:** Following the pre-operative instructions offered by the healthcare team is

critical to a successful operation. This might involve fasting before the surgery, stopping specific medicines, or performing pre-operative exams or assessments.

3. Prepare Your Home: Make the necessary preparations at home to provide a pleasant and secure rehabilitation environment. This may include creating a specific rehabilitation room with easy access to critical goods, arranging for help with daily duties, and adapting the home environment to meet mobility demands.

4. Maintaining a good mindset may have a big influence on the healing process. While it is natural to have times of uncertainty or frustration, concentrating on the progress accomplished and keeping hopeful about the future will help you stay motivated and resilient.

5. Don't Rush Recovery: Allow plenty of time for relaxation and recuperation after surgery. It's important to listen to your body and avoid pushing yourself too hard too quickly. Follow your healthcare team's recommendations about activity limitations and gradually increase physical activity as tolerated.

6. Stay Connected: Maintain contact with family, friends, and healthcare professionals throughout the healing process. Having a support structure in place may help give encouragement, motivation, and emotional support during difficult times.

Importance Of A Support System During Recovery

The support of family, friends, and healthcare professionals is critical in the healing process after spinal fusion surgery. A solid support system may provide emotional encouragement, practical aid, and important direction on the road to recovery.

Emotional Support:

1. Understanding and Empathy: Loved ones who provide understanding and empathy may assist in alleviating the emotional weight of healing. Having someone to speak to about your worries, concerns, and disappointments may bring comfort and reassurance at difficult times.

2. Positive support and inspiration from family and friends may help patients keep focused on their rehabilitation objectives. Celebrating milestones, no matter how modest, may raise morale and provide a feeling of achievement.

Practical Assistance:

1. **Assistance with Daily Tasks:** After surgery, patients may need assistance with daily chores such as cooking, cleaning, or errands. Family members or caregivers who provide practical support might help patients relax and heal.

2. **Transportation and movement Support:** After surgery, patients may have limited movement, making transportation difficult. Family members or friends who provide transportation to medical visits or

physical therapy sessions might help to maintain continuity of treatment and encourage recovery.

Guidance and advocacy:

1. Navigating the Healthcare System: The healing process after spinal fusion surgery may entail many healthcare providers and visits. Having a loved one who can assist the patient navigate the healthcare system, connect with clinicians, and advocate for their needs may guarantee complete treatment and the best possible results.

2. Information and services: Family members and caregivers may help patients learn about the operation, recovery process, and accessible services. This might entail looking into post-operative workouts, arranging for medical equipment, or contacting community support agencies.

The support of family, friends, and healthcare professionals is crucial throughout the healing period after spinal fusion surgery.

A robust support system may help patients traverse the hurdles of rehabilitation and achieve success by offering emotional encouragement, practical aid, and direction. Patients must freely explain their requirements and seek help from their support network as necessary. Patients who have the support of loved ones and healthcare professionals may overcome barriers and go on a road of healing and recovery.

CHAPTER 10

Future Developments And Advances

Emerging Technologies And Techniques In Spinal Surgery

Advances in medical technology continue to transform the landscape of spinal surgery, providing patients with more options and better results. One major advance is the development of less invasive surgical methods. Unlike typical open operations, which need large incisions and severe tissue damage, minimally invasive techniques use specialized equipment and imaging technologies to reach the spine via tiny incisions. This method minimizes stress to adjacent tissues, resulting in faster recovery durations, less postoperative discomfort, and a reduced chance of problems.

Another intriguing area of advancement is the use of robots in spinal surgery. Robotic-assisted systems increase surgeons' accuracy and control during surgeries, resulting in more precise implant placement and better surgical results. By combining modern imaging technologies with robotic guiding systems, surgeons may traverse complicated anatomical structures more easily and confidently, resulting in improved patient outcomes and a lower risk of problems.

In addition to technical developments, there is an increasing interest in the use of biologics in spine surgery. Biologics, such as stem cells and growth factors, have the potential to stimulate tissue regeneration and repair, providing novel treatments for degenerative disc disease, spinal cord injuries, and other spinal disorders. While research in this field is continuing, preliminary findings indicate that biologics may play an important role in the future of spinal surgery by improving healing and long-term outcomes for patients.

Overall, the future of spine surgery seems promising, with newer technology and procedures providing new opportunities to improve patient care and results. There is optimism for improved treatment choices for those suffering from spinal problems, including less invasive treatments, robotic-assisted surgery, and the use of biologics.

Possible Future Treatments For Spinal Conditions

As our knowledge of spinal diseases evolves, researchers are looking for novel therapy options to address the underlying causes and improve patient outcomes. Gene therapy might be used in the future to address genetic defects linked with certain spinal illnesses. Gene therapy, which delivers therapeutic genes directly to afflicted cells, can fix underlying genetic flaws and prevent disease development, providing fresh hope for those suffering from illnesses including spinal muscular atrophy and hereditary spine disorders.

Another area of study is the development of tissue engineering techniques for spinal cord repair. Tissue engineering is the process of generating specialized cells on scaffolds or matrices that have the same structure and function as natural tissues. Researchers hope to encourage regeneration and restore function by implanting these synthetic tissues into the wounded spinal cord, opening up new options for those who have suffered spinal cord injuries.

In addition to these innovative techniques, researchers are investigating the use of tailored medication delivery devices to treat spinal disorders. Researchers can precisely regulate the delivery of medications to particular parts of the spine by encapsulating them in biocompatible materials such as nanoparticles or hydrogels, therefore reducing adverse effects and increasing therapeutic effectiveness.

Overall, the future of spinal condition therapies seems promising, with continuous research opening the way for novel techniques to improve patient outcomes and quality of life. Gene therapy and tissue engineering, as well as tailored medication delivery systems, provide promise for improved treatment choices for those suffering from spine disorders.

The Importance Of Research And Innovation In Improving Surgical Results

Research and innovation are critical to advancing spinal surgery and increasing patient outcomes. By constantly pushing the frontiers of medical knowledge and technology, researchers and clinicians may create new methods, improve current procedures, and uncover novel therapies for spinal disorders.

Research leads to better surgical results by improving our knowledge of the spine's biomechanics. Researchers who investigate the intricate connections between the many components of the spine may create more successful surgical procedures and implant designs that better replicate the spine's natural function, resulting in greater stability and long-term results for patients.

In addition to biomechanics, research is critical to the advancement of imaging technology, which is required for planning and carrying out spine procedures. Researchers can provide surgeons with detailed, real-time images of the spine by developing more advanced imaging modalities such as MRI and CT scans, allowing for more precise preoperative planning and intraoperative navigation, resulting in better surgical outcomes and a lower risk of complications.

Furthermore, research encourages innovation in surgical instruments and technology, allowing surgeons to conduct treatments more precisely and efficiently. From robotic-assisted surgery systems to minimally invasive surgical equipment, advances in surgical technology are transforming the field of spine surgery, opening up new avenues for enhancing patient care and results.

Overall, research and innovation play a very important role in improving surgical results. By encouraging cooperation among clinicians, researchers, and industry partners, we may continue to push the frontiers of spinal surgery and discover novel solutions that enhance patient outcomes and quality of life.

Hope For Better Options For People With Spinal Issues

Despite the difficulties that spinal problems provide, there is hope for those who suffer from them. New treatment alternatives are developing as a result of continuous research and technological breakthroughs, with the potential to improve patient outcomes and quality of life.

One source of optimism is the increased focus on customized treatment in spinal care. Clinicians may improve results and reduce the risk of problems by adapting treatment techniques to each patient's unique requirements and features. From modern imaging methods to genetic testing and biomarker analysis, customized medicine has the potential to transform how spinal illnesses are identified and treated, providing fresh hope to those affected.

In addition to individualized medicine, there is rising interest in interdisciplinary methods of spinal care that entail cooperation across multiple specialists, including neurosurgery, orthopedic surgery, physical therapy, and pain management. Multidisciplinary care teams may create complete treatment regimens that meet the varied requirements of patients with spinal disorders, resulting in better outcomes and quality of life.

Furthermore, advances in regenerative medicine and tissue engineering have the potential to benefit those suffering from spinal cord injuries and degenerative disc diseases. Researchers hope to boost tissue regeneration and repair by tapping into the body's inherent healing systems, opening up new options for restoring function and enhancing mobility in those with spinal difficulties.

Overall, although spinal diseases pose considerable obstacles, there is hope for improved solutions in the future. We can enhance the lives of those suffering from spinal problems by continuing to study, innovate, and collaborate.

Conclusion

Knowing spinal fusion surgery entails comprehending its aim, technique, dangers, advantages, and healing process. This detailed guide delves into the complexities of this frequent surgical surgery designed to stabilize the spine, relieve pain, and improve the overall quality of life for patients suffering from spinal problems.

Spinal fusion surgery is a critical treatment for a variety of spinal conditions, including degenerative disc disease, spinal stenosis, spondylolisthesis, and spinal fractures. The treatment involves fusing two or more vertebrae to limit mobility at the afflicted section, therefore lowering discomfort and avoiding additional damage to the spinal cord and nerves.

Throughout the course, we've looked at the various surgical methods used in spinal fusion, from standard open surgery to less invasive treatments. Each procedure has benefits and disadvantages, and the decision is based on criteria such as the patient's health, the surgeon's preference, and technological advances.

However, spinal fusion surgery has several risks and problems, such as infection, blood clots, nerve injury, and failed fusion. Patients must be informed of these possible consequences and communicate openly with their healthcare professionals to reduce risks and increase their chances of success.

Despite the inherent hazards, spinal fusion surgery provides significant advantages, including pain alleviation, greater spinal stability, more mobility, and a higher quality of life. However, it is critical to establish realistic expectations and recognize that complete recovery may take many months, including physical therapy, lifestyle changes, and adherence to postoperative instructions.

Furthermore, the choice to have spinal fusion surgery should be made collaboratively by patients, their families, and healthcare experts. A thorough examination, education, and exploration of alternative treatment alternatives are critical for making educated choices that are consistent with the patient's objectives and desires.

In summary, spinal fusion surgery is an important step in treating spinal diseases, but it is not a one-size-fits-all cure. Each patient's condition is unique, and treatment options should be customized to their specific requirements and circumstances.

Finally, this book is an excellent resource for anybody looking to get a thorough grasp of spinal fusion surgery. By providing patients with information and insights, we want to support informed decision-making, effective communication with healthcare professionals, and, ultimately, better results and experiences for people undergoing this revolutionary treatment.

THE END

www.ingramcontent.com/pod-product-compliance
Lightning Source LLC
Chambersburg PA
CBHW061245250726

48653CB00002B/524